GW01048800

EXTREME MILITARY FITNESS

BASIC

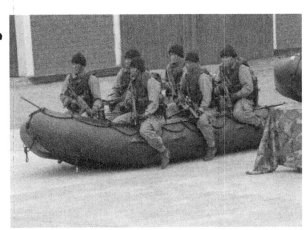

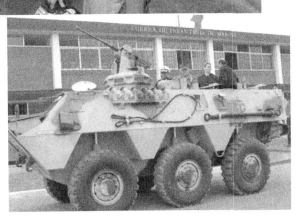

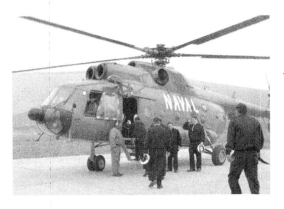

USING THE BEST OF AMERICAN, ISRAELI AND RUSSIAN MILITARY TRAINING METHODS TO FORGE A NEW YOU!

BY

ERIC GUTTMANN

EXTREME MILITARY FITNESS

BASIC

USING THE BEST OF AMERICAN, ISRAELI AND RUSSIAN MILITARY TRAINING METHODS TO FORGE A NEW YOU!

BY

ERIC GUTTMANN

An Eric Guttmann Book / Original Copyright Eric Guttmann Enterprises, Inc. © March 2009

All rights reserved.

No part of this book may be reproduced or transmitted in any form or by any means, electronic or mechanical, including photocopying, recording, or by any informational storage and retrieval system, without permission from the publisher.

Guttmann, Inc.
P.O. Box 330245
Atlantic Beach, FL 32233

Disclaimer

The exercises and advice within this book may be too strenuous or dangerous for some people, and the reader(s) should consult a physician before engaging in them.

The author and publisher of this book are not responsible in any manner whatsoever for any injury which may occur through reading and following the instructions herein

Dedication

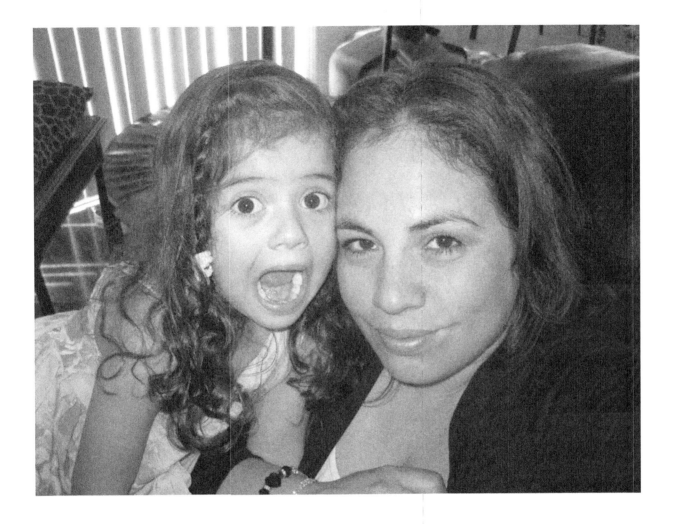

I dedicate this course to my wife Vianca, who was the first person to see the potential and to have the wisdom to tell me *"What you need to do is stop buying all these other courses and start writing one of your own!"* Thank you for believing in me! I also dedicate this course to my daughter Vianca Patricia for always barging into my workouts and demanding to exercise with me as well!

WHAT PEOPLE ARE SAYING ABOUT EXTREME MILITARY FITNESS

"What I love about this course is Eric's intensity of attitude and achievement. He begins where we all begin – at the bottom of physical development. He then brings us step by step to an impressive level of athletic conditioning. EXTREME MILITARY FITNESS will take you to levels you'll be pleasantly surprised with. Yes, levels you didn't think you could attain! I highly recommend my friend Eric's book and course!"
Peter Ragnar
Author of over 25 life-changing books and courses
www.roaringlionpublishing.com

"Move over, P90X®! Naval Officer Eric Guttmann uses his skills as a certified Elite Combat Fitness Instructor to create a new program that makes **Extreme Military Fitness** available to all who truly desire it. This no-nonsense program combines common exercises in uncommon ways to provide you the warrior's level of conditioning that you have always wanted."
Eddie Armstrong
Wisdom of the Mystic Mountain Warrior
Available at www.roaringlionpublishing.com

"Eric Guttmann has put together a simple yet effective program combining two of my favorite ways to train, kettlebells and bodyweight exercises. And he has taken the guesswork out of it by making it seriously step by step. You add the effort and you will get the result."
Logan Christopher
The Definitive Guide to Kettlebell Juggling
www.kettlebelljuggling.com

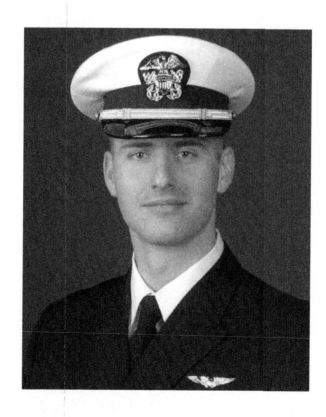

READ THIS FIRST

Dear Friend,

Congratulations on your purchase of Extreme Military Fitness Level 1. You now have in your hands a complete blueprint to achieve functional fitness using the military training secrets of the Americans, Israelis and Russians.

Consider this your indoctrination into the world of functional fitness.

Your training begins today!

Perhaps it will be useful to let you know the very first set of orders I received upon arriving at the U.S. Navy's Officer Candidate School in Pensacola, Florida: "From now on the only reply you will give to any question is 'Yes Sir!', 'No Sir" or 'No Excuse Sir!' Is that understood?"

I urge you to adopt that same attitude towards your training.

Why train with Bodyweight Exercises and Kettlebells?

There is a quote from Thucydides, the famous Greek historian and author of the *History of the Peloponnesian War* between Athens and Sparta, that has influenced me a lot. This quote is that "We must remember that one man is much the same as another, and that he is best who is trained in the severest school."

Inside every one of us there is the person we wish to become. For some people it is their untrained and undisciplined bodies that hold them back from achieving their true and wonderful potential.

It is no secret that the American, Israeli and Russian militaries have produced some of the finest and toughest soldiers of the modern age. The more elite the unit, the more Spartan zeal is displayed in every aspect of training.

This leads us to how these militaries have gotten their soldiers to peak physical performance levels. Was it with bodybuilding workouts and supplements? No. The answer was with good old fashioned functional bodyweight exercises for both the American and Israeli forces, and with kettlebells for the Russians.

To truly depend on your body to carry you to victory in extreme circumstances requires a lot more than the ability to lift heavy weights. This program is the realization of that fact and how I learned what I REALLY needed to do to be fit.

Another quote from Thucydides which I learned while stationed at the Naval Postgraduate School that has affected how I view the world is the account of the Melian dialogue.

During the Peloponnesian War, the Athenians were looking to annex the island of Melos. Discussions where held between the Athenians and the Melians. The Athenians gave the Melians two options: submit and live or fight and die. The Melians expressed a desire for neutrality and started talking about justice. The Athenians, who were the stronger of the two, bluntly told the Melians, "You know as well as we do that in this world, justice is a subject for debate only among those who are equals in power. The strong do what they can and the weak suffer what they must." The Melians refused to submit and were wiped out.

Now while this phrase has been used to explain what is called the Realist perspective in the study of international relations, the key point I PERSONALLY draw from it is that we should do all we can to BE STRONG and do all we can to avoid being weak! This program will show you how.

I recommend you read through the whole manual first, watch the Bodyweight DVD second and finish with the Kettlebell DVD. This is the surest way to understanding.

One more thing, you will note that there is a slight image distortion in some of the pictures in this manual, specifically with the burpee illustrations, as my intent was to get them all in ONE page. It is by focusing on the information that the pictures seek to transmit rather than their quality that you will get the most our of this course. This combined with the DVD instruction should leave you with a clear and crisp idea of how to properly perform every exercise in this book.

The strength and conditioning that you get from this course is transferable and will help you to accomplish other training programs with ease. Here I am making a partial deadlift with 14 plates on the bar after getting Peter Ragnar's Serious Strength course. Remember there is no ONE way to train! There are multiple ways to train and they all bring about different results.

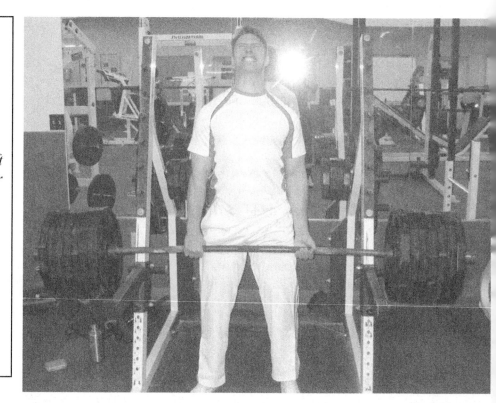

THE PROGRAM

This program is designed to get you in the best functional combat ready shape of your life in 12 weeks. You will learn and implement the tools and techniques that have been proven to turn ordinary citizens into highly disciplined fighting units.

This program is strict but fair. For some of you there will be a steep learning curve as you see some or all of the exercises for the first time. For others you will get reacquainted with old "friends". Incorporated into the program is enough time to learn and to MASTER these exercises. In mastering the workouts you are mastering yourself.

As a US Naval Officer and an Elite Combat Fitness instructor I have distilled for you the very best of what I know into a streamlined program of functional fitness that will be easy to understand and challenging to perform.

Let's be clear. You may or may not be in the best shape of your life right now. It does not matter. The alternating program of bodyweight and ketllebell workouts you are about to embark on will help you to achieve an awesome level of FUNCTIONAL fitness regardless of where you are at today.

Regardless of your current level of conditioning is, this program will WORK for you! The program has a gradual introduction that allows you to build up to the level of fitness desired.

You WILL perform 48 workouts, 4 workouts per week, over the course of the next 12 weeks. I respect your time, so your workouts will NOT go over 30 minutes. You WILL alternate between bodyweight workouts and kettlebell circuits for a total of two bodyweight and two kettlebell workouts a week.

Look if I had to add up every seminar I have attended, every certification I have, every book I have read and every DVD I own to bring you this document, this blueprint, then you are looking at close to $10,000 of my own money and hundreds of hours of trial and error finding out what works and what doesn't.

When I read something regarding human performance, my first thought is "Oh yeah, let's PROVE it!" I invite you to adopt the same attitude and attack this training program with the attitude of "prove to me it works!" The way you do that is by sticking with it for 12 weeks and doing all 48 workouts before you make your final judgment. I am confident that you will be both surprised and amazed at the person you will become at the end of those 12 weeks.

I can't wait to read all your success stories!

MY STORY

The 98 pound weakling

You know how some people are born strong and athletic and everything seems to be working out for them physically, well that was not me.

I was clumsy, uncoordinated and weak. This meant that I was always picked last in gym class, even after the girls. In today's day and age there is no shame in this, but back in 1980 it was an embarrassment for a guy to be picked after all the girls were divvied up. That trend of being the last guy picked in gym class continued all throughout grade school.

In junior high the jocks would always pick on the least developed and less talented on the field and that would be me. I thought to myself, "these guys are a bunch of assholes," and I made a decision right then and there to never pick on anybody because they were weaker than me. On the contrary, I would help them out, because I knew how it felt to be the one nobody wants.

While I knew I never wanted to be like them I did want to stop being a weakling.

In 7th grade we had some tests involving 1 minute of push ups and situps, and I could not do a single push up!

I got in the position and started to go down, but could *not* push back up. My trembling hands just gave way and my body hit the floor of the gym.

I got 0 pushups for that 1 minute test. That's right, z-e-r-o, I failed it. That was a big blow.

So finally I got pissed off and I just started to work out in my room by doing push ups against the dresser drawer, since I could not do them against the floor.

That was my own little secret. Nobody knew what I was doing.

I would do as many pushups as I could everyday at this 45 degree angle.

After two months I tried to do a pushup against the floor and failed miserably, so I again hit the dresser drawer with a vengeance. After two more months I tried again and I was finally able to do five pushups. I was ecstatic.

I was able to do my first pushup at the age of 12. This was a huge deal for me!

Learning to workout in a REAL gym and the U.S. Army

When I was 14 I joined a gym. Not just any gym, but a HARDCORE gym. Forget the aerobic classes and tight leotards, this was a DUNGEON. I am talking about professional bodybuilders, wrestlers, bouncers, DEA Agents, Customs Agents, ex-military, airport personnel and skinny, fourteen year old ME. These men of iron became my surrogate fathers of strength.

From the time I was 14 to 18 I did not get picked on by the jocks or other classmates and people generally gave me a respectful deference because of my size and strength. I even joined the U.S. Army and became a journalist and Public Affairs Specialist with the 65th Regional Support Command in Fort Buchanan, PR. The strength and work ethic I had forged in the gym helped me to become a Non-Commissioned Officer within four years and Soldier of the Year in 1998.

I kept on working out and by the time I was 23 I could already bench press 315lbs.

So after finishing my undergraduate in Education and with my commitment to the U.S. Army done, I had the freedom to forge my own path now. I was learning Chen Style Taijiquan and I asked my instructor what were the keys to be good in this art. He said, "all great practitioners of Taijiquan are well versed in Chinese Medicine." Therefore I went to New York to work on my masters in Acupuncture and Oriental Medicine.

The U.S. Navy

Then 9/11 happened and I knew that I wanted to go back in the military and do my part. I felt that I needed to do something to provide a more secure world for my children to grow up in.

I ended up flying for the Navy.

Back in the military I attacked the culture of fitness with a vengeance. Since I had to be in shape to serve my country, I was constantly reading, implementing and experimenting with what works and doesn't regarding health, fitness, workouts and performance.

I went to Officer Candidate School in Pensacola, Florida, got commissioned and then continued to earn my navy wings of gold in Randolph Air Force Base in San Antonio, TX.

After that I went to Survival, Evasion, Resistance and Escape (SERE) training in Brunswick, Maine.

Now, if you saw the movie G.I. Jane and remember the prison camp scene, that is SERE school. While that was a movie with a lot of exaggerations, we are not allowed to divulge information about the training and therefore cannot set the record straight.

All I can say is that it was the most realistic training American service members can go through to prepare for and EXPERIENCE the eventuality of being captured by a ruthless enemy and being able to return with honor and we all had return tickets home.

Unlike our brothers and sisters who have had to pay the ultimate sacrifice, we knew we were in a training environment.

Flying for the Navy!

After SERE school I went to the final phase of my training in Naval Air Station Whidbey Island where I learned about Electronic Warfare. Now I was ready to report to my first operational squadron, Fleet Air Reconnaissance Squadron Two in Rota, Spain.

Operationally, I deployed four times to the Middle East, twice to the Far East and once to the Mediterranean. While I can't really talk about what we do, there are some sea stories I can recall…

Iran? What do you mean we are going to fly over Iran?

I was flying overland Iraq in 2007 when I was training an up and coming Naval Officer for the position of Senior Evaluator (SEVAL) on the EP-3 Signals Intelligence Reconnaissance Aircraft.

I allowed him to sit in "the seat" of the SEVAL while I watched from behind.

While running his systems cross check, in this case the aircraft's position by checking the Global Positioning System to the computer mission system, he nervously looked at me and said "I think we are 20 miles off course, what do we do?"

Now, this was a big deal. You don't want to be the one who stops the mission if you are wrong; however, there is only a five mile corridor when leaving Iraq and if you are 20 miles off course you can easily fly into Iranian airspace. That would be a very bad thing.

So he was right in being concerned.

One quick glance at his map screen confirmed my suspicion that his technique was a little off.

He had zoomed out so much that a tiny error in cursor placement showed a huge amount of distance.

In other words, if you were half an inch off, that would easily translate into 20 miles.

I told him to zoom in the picture and do the cross check again. He did this and breathed a sigh of relief as he let me know that we had a good cross check. I did not broadcast his rookie error to the whole crew by correcting his mistake before anyone noticed.

Hey, that's what I was there for.

The price of freedom

In aviation we have a sterile cockpit environment. When we fly we talk to the same guys over a period of time and you build a relationship with a "voice" over the radios.

However, when you are flying and you hear their callsign followed by the letters K-I-A, which stand for Killed-In-Action, you get this sinking feeling in the pit of your stomach and all your hairs stand on end.

That's a guy with a family who just made his wife a widow and whose kids just became orphans.

That's the guy who may have just worked out with you in the gym, or with whom you just shared a meal with in the galley.

That was a reminder that it could have been me and that nothing in this life is guaranteed.

Bring him back alive!

While flying operations in the Middle East I also got an opportunity to be a Liaison Naval Officer working in the Combined Air Operations Center in Southwest Asia. My main job was to assign planes to missions in support of Operation Iraqi Freedom.

At the end of a twelve hour day you just want to go home. I will never forget the energy in the room when we had notification that an emergency beacon went off on the ground in Iraq.

One of our guys needed help!

We were going to initiate a Personal Recovery effort.

Right then and there every single one of us, even though tired and ready to go home to sleep from a long day only a few seconds ago, suddenly became alive and was ready to do all they could to help out. Having a well trained and disciplined body that can handle extra hours of important work at the END of a long day is extremely important.

We all wanted to get our guy back alive!

And yes, eventually we got our guy back, in fact my wife's cousin was in the unit that recovered him. It's a small world.

My operational tour provided me with the opportunity to be an Operations Mission Statistics Officer, Ground Safety Officer and a Tactics Division Officer on top of being a SEVAL in Fleet Air Reconnaissance Squadron Two with over 970 hours, flying over 125 operational missions including 42 combat missions supporting Operation Iraqi Freedom.

I would not trade that experience for anything in the world!

Commando Krav Maga and Elite Combat Fitness

During my military career I kept on training and achieved some of my personal bests, which include bench pressing 365lbs, squatting 405lbs and deadlifting 350lbs.

I was doing this in my spare time while flying missions, getting qualified and having a family with four kids.

So when I joined a Commando Krav Maga class I thought I would be ready for anything they threw at me.

That was until I learned that the warm up would consist of a series of exercises called Elite Combat Fitness which were developed by Moni Aizik, a former member of the Israeli Special Forces Elite Commando Unit. These exercises combine high caliber Olympic conditioning drills, exercises used by Mixed Martial Arts fighters, and challenging military routines used by Elite Commandos.

A humbling experience!

I kept a straight face throughout the class, but inside my body was screaming "Please make it stop!"

I suddenly realized that I was not as fit as I thought I was and that all my strength training was not worth as much when it came to functional strength and conditioning. Not to mention the fact that all the heavy lifts, while making me stronger, where taking their toll on my shoulders, elbows and hips.

After one month of training and feeling way out of my league, I took a bold step.

I signed up for the Elite Combat Fitness Instructor course!

I could have just quit the class to avoid being faced with reality and just headed back to the gym to lift more iron...but I knew I had just stumbled unto something more powerful than just weight training!

The Elite Combat Fitness instructor course was in fact the most physically demanding and humbling experience I have ever undertaken in my life - and I have been through Army Boot Camp, Navy Officer Candidate School, SERE school, graduated from the naval aviation pipeline and flown over 125 Combat Reconnaissance Missions, 42 of them overland Iraq!

To become an instructor you had to survive three grueling days of non stop exercise. You learned and PERFORMED every exercise and workout routine in the Elite Combat Fitness manual. This includes the staple of military training like squats, burpees, pushups, mountain climbers, as well as single, partner and group workouts, log drills, uphill runs, outdoor courses, the suicide mission, and also introduced us to the Russian kettlebell, which is basically a cannonball with a handle attached to it. After becoming and instructor I really wanted to put this system to the test.

So I stopped all weightlifting and running and did nothing but a unique combination of drills for my Physical Readiness Test. After four months of this type of training, without running a single day in those four months, I not only maxed my situps and pushups, but shaved 15 seconds off my run.

And I lost 10 lbs to boot without really trying, all the while raiding the kids snacks at night! This leads us to training and the power of a coach.

The power of a coach and mentor

That's where I can try to help you. I am not going to ask you to do anything I have not personally done myself. I know from experience this program works.

No one succeeds alone. I would like to give you the same assurance I gave my trainee flying overland Iraq. By joining the ranks of Extreme Military Fitness, I will be standing behind you as you work towards your goals.

When I tell you that my program worked for me and it can work for you it's because it DOES!

A Naval Officer's word is his bond. You can expect my program and me to stay the course as you work diligently towards your fitness goals.

If you don't quit on me, I won't quit on you!

WHAT YOU CAN EXPECT FROM EXTREME MILITARY FITNESS LEVEL 1:

1. Achieve combat ready physical fitness levels and burn fat a lot faster. I lost ten pounds without trying!

2. Only 6 minutes a week on pushups on average.

3. Radically increase your endurance inside 90 days and have boundless energy to get everything you need to get done through the day.

4. Only 12 minutes a week of abdominal work on average.

5. Train your mind and body to perform on demand!

6. Turn back the clock and look years younger as you do something to counteract obesity, poor heart conditions, high blood pressure and other deadly diseases that are afflicting today's population as a result of stress, poor eating habits and a lack of exercise.

7. No gym required (one Kettlebell or dumbbell, 35lb for men and 24lb for women will be required).

8. 4 workouts a week, each under 30 minutes.

9. No fat loss or bodybuilding supplements required, save your money and your health!

10. No need for a single running workout, save your joints!

11. Can be done alone or with a partner.

OK, I am already excited! Let's get to work!

BODYWEIGHT EXERCISES

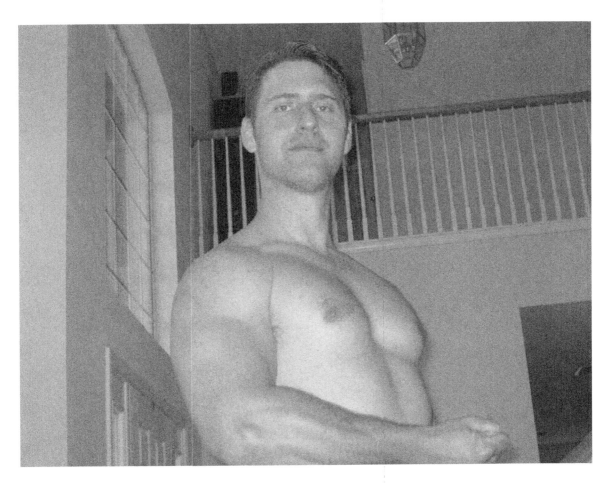

YOU CAN ACHIEVE A WARRIOR'S BODY FROM BODYWEIGHT EXERCISES!

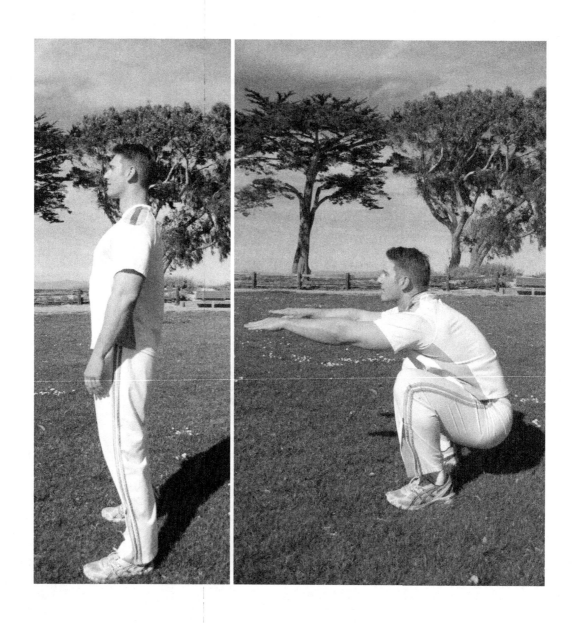

SLO-MO SQUAT

1. Start with your feet shoulder apart, looking forward, hands at your side.

2. Slo-o-o-w-l-y go down into the squat as you inhale and start counting to ten.

3. Your arms start reaching out as you go down for balance.

4. You should reach the bottom of the movement on the count of ten (one thousand one, one thousand two, …one thousand ten) with arms fully extended.

5. Exhale and slowly count to ten in the same manner as you push off with your heels and straighten up.

6. Hands slowly come towards the body.

7. At the count of ten you should be back at the starting position with hands at your side.

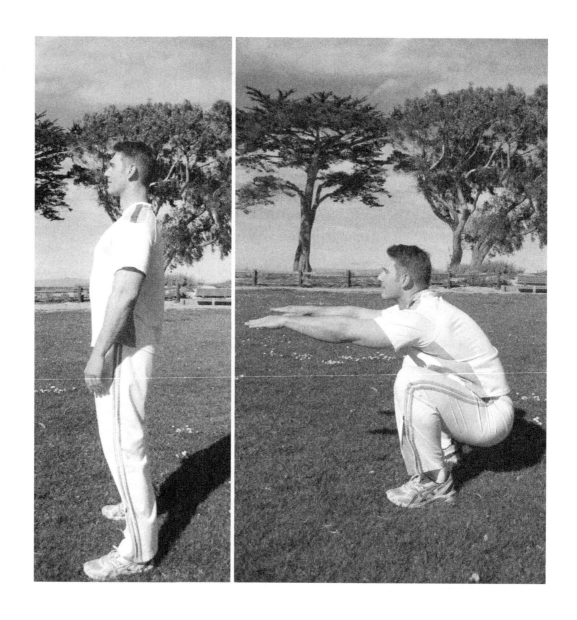

SQUAT

1. Start with your feet shoulder apart, looking forward, hands at your side.

2. Inhale as you go down.

3. Your arms start reaching out as you go down for balance.

4. You should reach the bottom of the movement with arms fully outstretched. You should go down to the count of one and come back up to the count of one. Instead of 20 seconds per rep as in the slo-mo squat, now aim for two seconds per rep.

5. Exhale as you explode up from your heels.

6. Hands come towards the body.

7. You are now in the starting position.

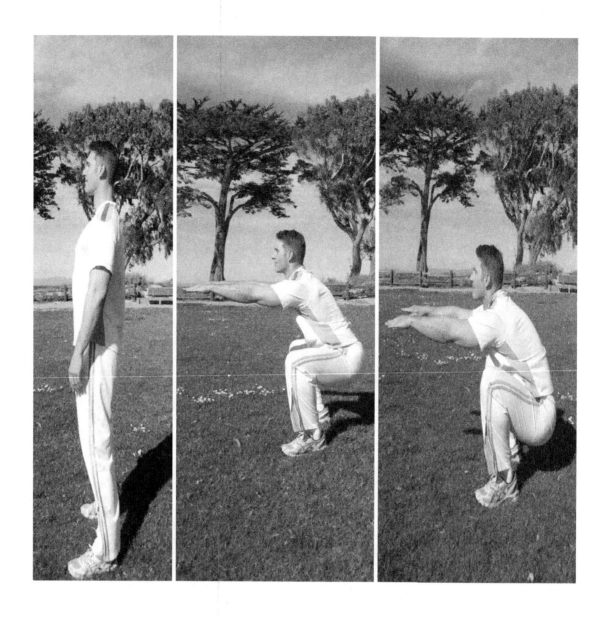

ABC SQUAT

Position A: standing upright, the starting position for squats
Position B: squat down to the halfway point so your knees are at 90 degree angle
Position C: squat down all the way, as low as your butt will go down

1.   Start with position A.

2.   Inhale as you go down to position B.

3.   Exhale as you explode into position A.

4.   Perform 10 repetitions.

5.   Inhale and go down into position C.

6.   Exhale as you explode into position B.

7.   Inhale as you return to position C.

8.   Perform 10 repetitions.

9.   Go to position A.

10.   Inhale as you go down to position C.

11.   Exhale as you explode into position A.

12.   Perform 10 repetitions.

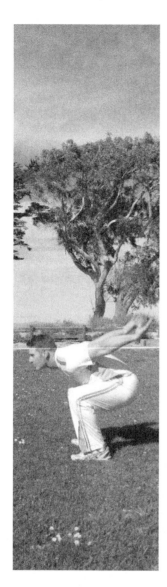
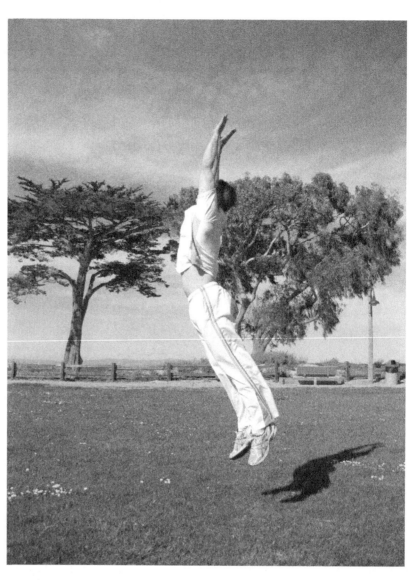

JUMP SQUAT

1. Start with your feet shoulder apart, looking forward, hands at your side.

2. Inhale as you go down.

3. Swing your arms behind you as you go down for momentum.

4. From the squat position, exhale and explode up in the air as you swing you hands up to get airborne.

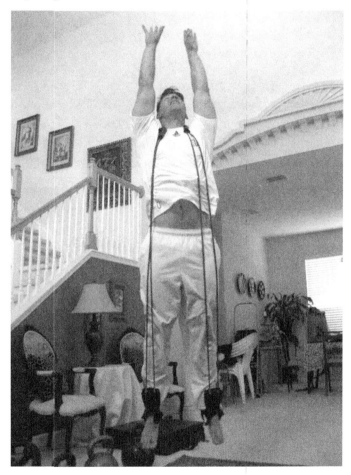

You can also try these with a Power Jumper to increase your explosive drive!

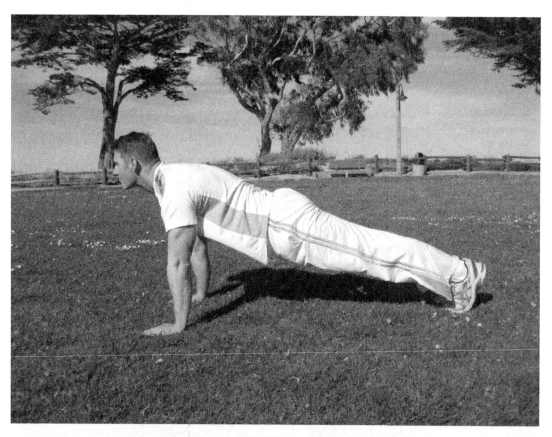

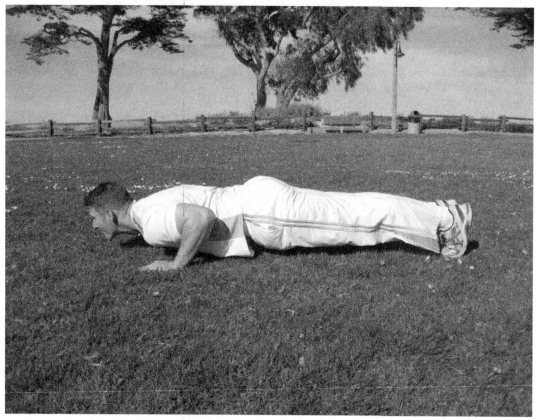

SLO-MO PUSHUP

1. Start with the pushup position with your hands shoulder width apart.

2. Inhale as you go down slo-o-o-o-wly with your elbows pointing towards your legs, aiming for a count of 10 on the way down (one thousand one, one thousand two, all the way to one thousand ten).

3. Exhale as you come up slo-o-o-o-wly aiming for a count of 10.

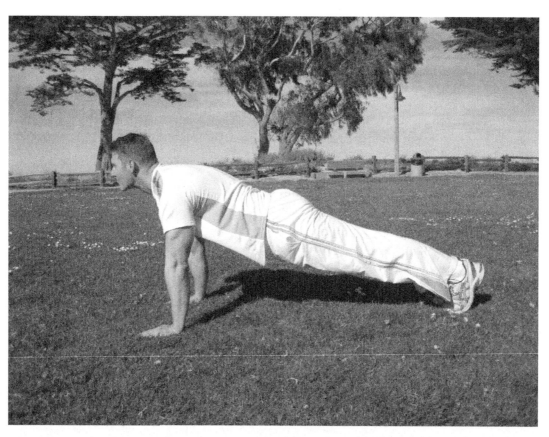

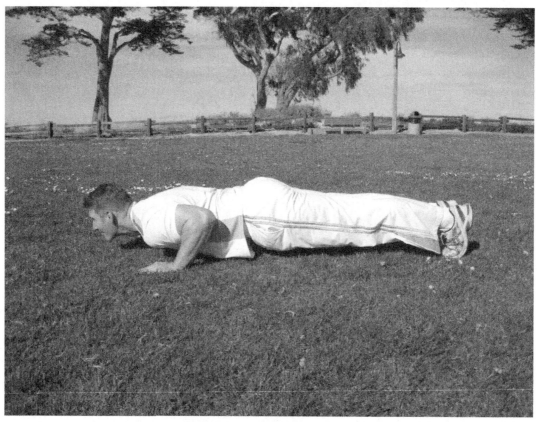

PUSHUP

1. Start with the pushup position with your hands shoulder width apart.

2. Inhale as you go down with your elbows pointing towards your legs.

3. Exhale as you explode up. As with the regular squat, aim for a two second repetition for the pushup, one second to go down and one second to come up.

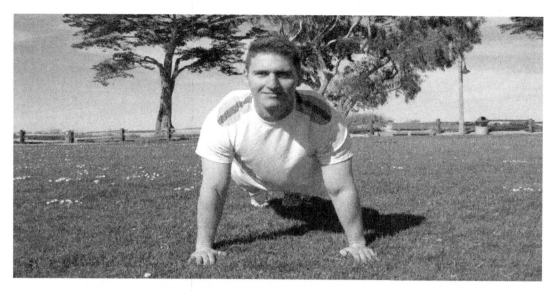

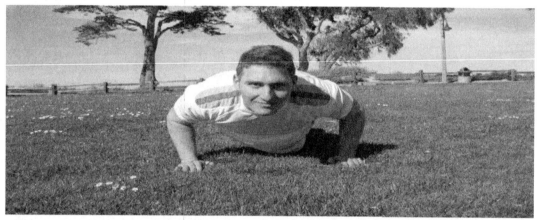

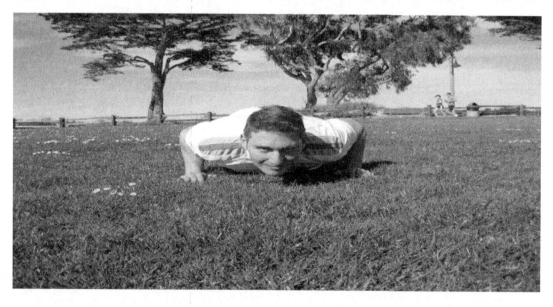

ABC PUSHUP

Position A: Regular pushup position
Position B: Halfway point of a pushup, elbows at 90 degrees
Position C: All the way down chest touching the ground

1. Start with position A.

2. Inhale as you go down to position B.

3. Exhale as you explode into position A.

4. Perform 10 repetitions.

5. Inhale and go down into position C.

6. Exhale as you explode into position B.

7. Inhale as you return to position C.

8. Perform 10 repetitions.

9. Go to position A.

10. Inhale as you go down to position C.

11. Exhale as you explode into position A.

12. Perform 10 repetitions.

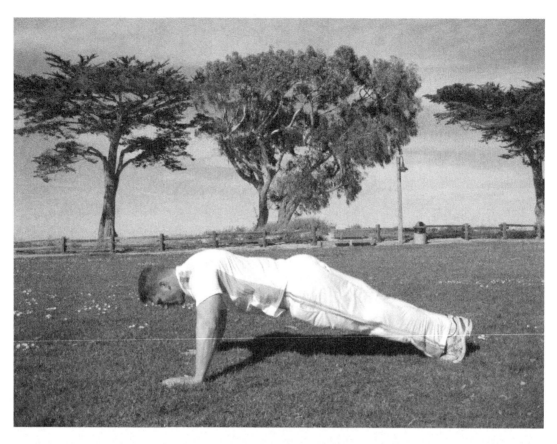

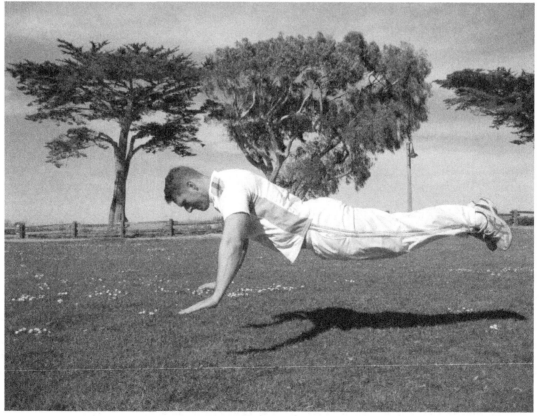

CLOCKWORK PUSHUP

1. Start with standard pushup position (this is the 12 o'clock position).

2. Inhale as you bend the arms, exhale as you EXPLODE the whole body into the air in a clockwise direction to the 1 o'clock position.

3. Keep on exploding clockwise until you cover all the hours of the clock (2, 3, 4, 5, 6, 7, 8, 9, 10, 11, 12).

4. After performing 12 repetitions, or one full turn clockwise, perform them counterclockwise.

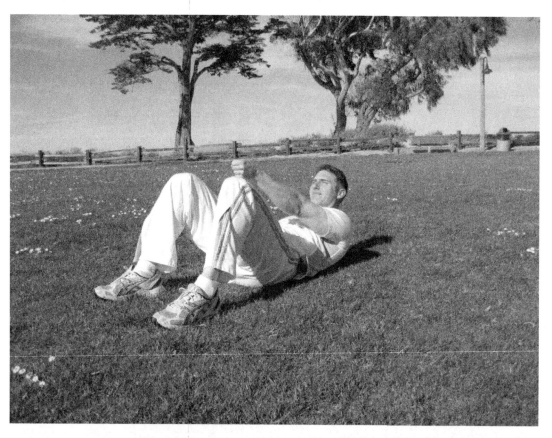

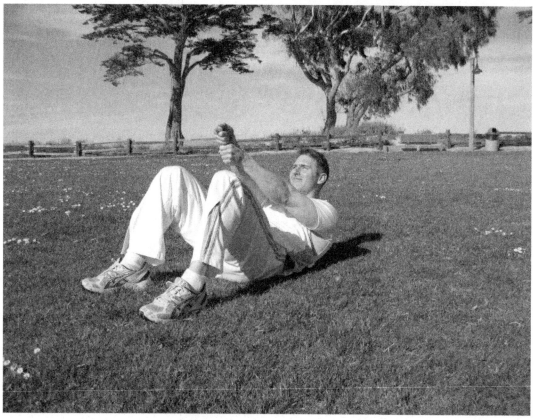

ROPE CRUNCH

1. Lie down on your back with knees bent.

2. Imagine pushing your bellybutton into the ground so that your lower back is pressing against the ground.

3. Slowly pull yourself up on an imaginary rope at a 45 degree angle towards the front (not straight up), aiming for 4-5 hand over hand passes.

4. At the top of the movement squeeze hard.

5. Come back down slowly with the same number of hand over hand passes.

6. If at any point your lower back stops touching the floor, re-engage by consciously pressing your bellybutton into the floor.

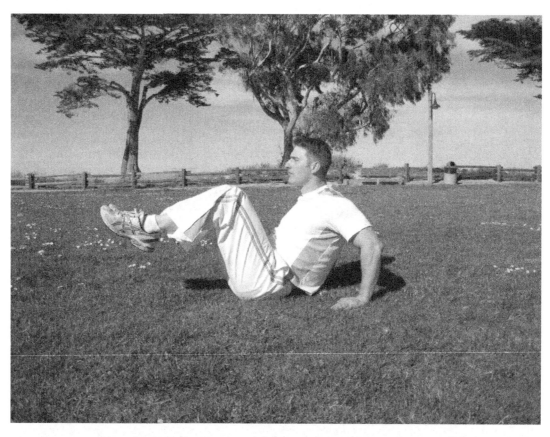

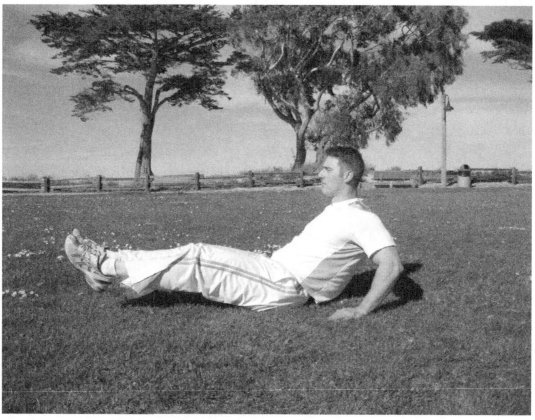

BENT LEG

JACKNIFE

1.   Lie down on the floor and place your hands behind your body.

2.   Raise your legs and find your balance point.

3.   Lean back with your hands helping you as your legs go forward.

4.   Contract and bring legs close to your body.

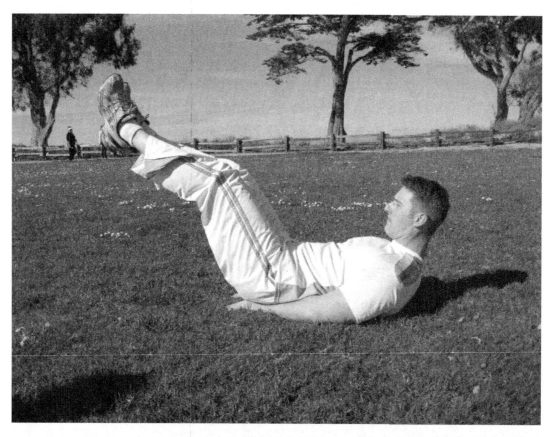

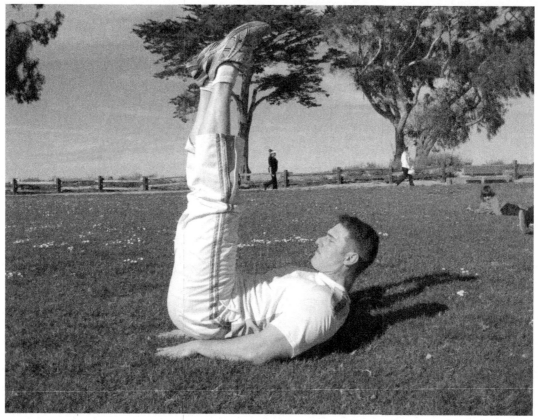

NEEDLE LIFT

1. Start lying flat on your back with your hands at your sides or under your glutes and legs at 45 degrees. Then bring your legs to 90 degrees towards the ceiling to begin the exercise.

2. Exhale as you slowly contract your lower abs and raise your legs towards the ceiling.

3. Inhale as you bring down your legs in a controlled manner to the starting position.

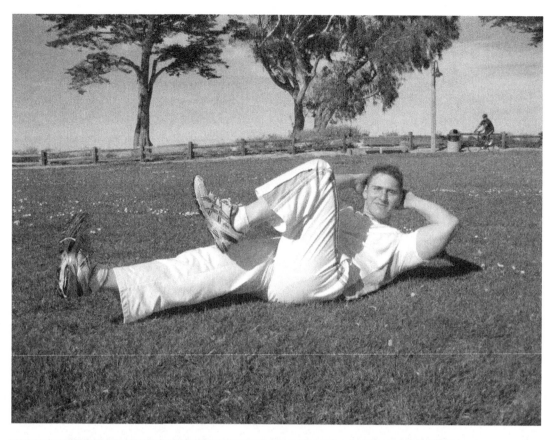

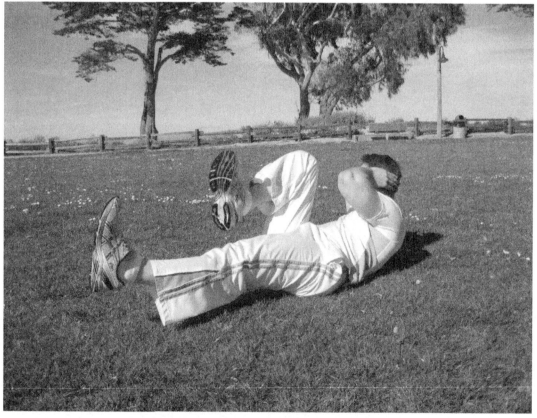

BICYCLE CRUNCHES

1. Lie on your back and bring one knee up to meet opposing elbow.

2. While keeping this crunch position switch to the other elbow and the opposing knee.

3. Pump your legs in and out, pressing with the heels.

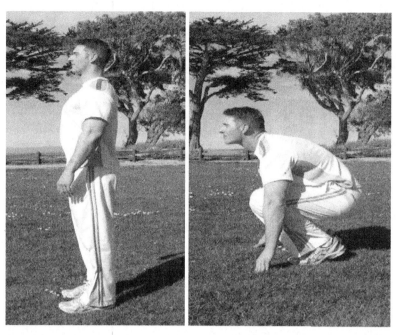

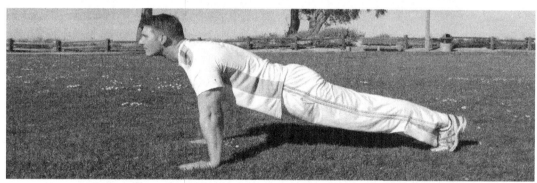

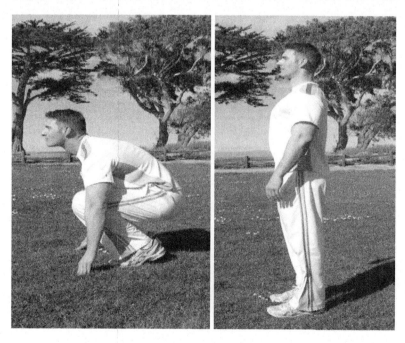

EASY BURPEE

1.   Start from a regular standing position.

2.   Inhale as you bend your knees into a tucked position.

3.   Exhale as you explode your legs out into the pushup position.

4.   Inhale as you bring your legs back to the tucked position.

5.   Exhale as you explode into the standing position.

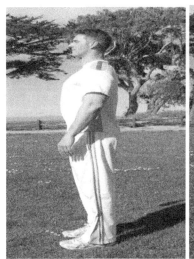
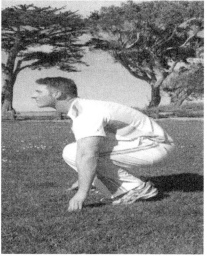

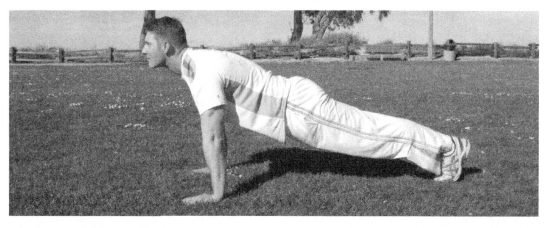

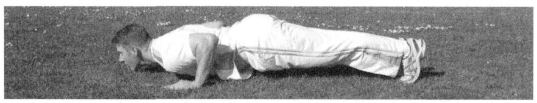

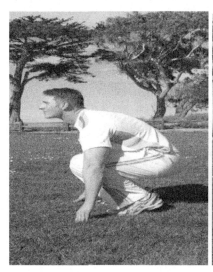
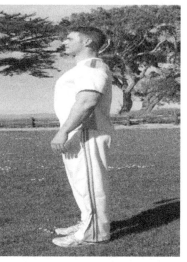

43

BURPEE WITH PUSHUP

1. Start from a regular standing position.

2. Inhale as you bend your knees into a tucked position.

3. Exhale as you explode your legs out into the pushup position.

4. Inhale as you go down to the ground.

5. Exhale as you explode into the pushup position.

6. Inhale as you bring your legs back to the tucked position.

7. Exhale as you explode into the standing position.

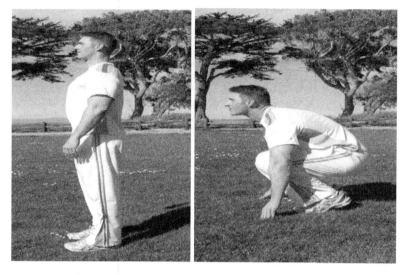

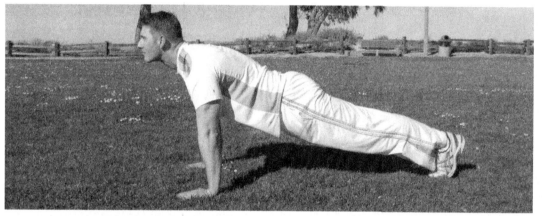

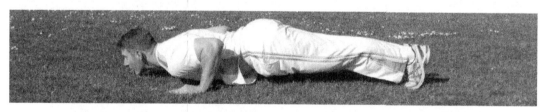

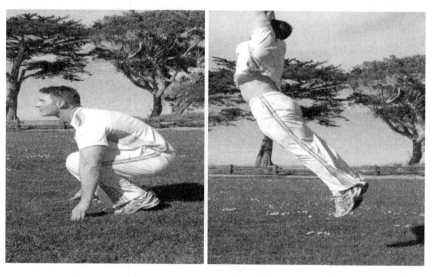

JUMP BURPEE

1. Start from a regular standing position.

2. Inhale as you bend your knees into a tucked position.

3. Exhale as you explode your legs out into the pushup position.

6. Inhale as you go down to the ground.

7. Exhale as you explode into the pushup position.

8. Inhale as you bring your legs back to the tucked position.

9. Exhale as you explode into the air while swinging your arms up.

"IF YOU DO SOMETHING EVERYDAY, THEN EVERYDAY YOU WILL BE ABLE TO DO IT."

-ENDRE GUTTMANN

MY FATHER SHARING SOME WISDOM HIS GRECO-ROMAN WRESTLING COACH IN HUNGARY GAVE HIM REGARDING PHYSICAL TRAINING.

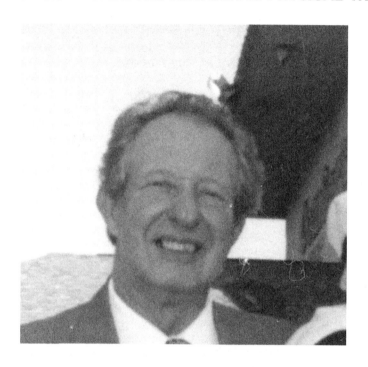

KETTLEBELL EXERCISES

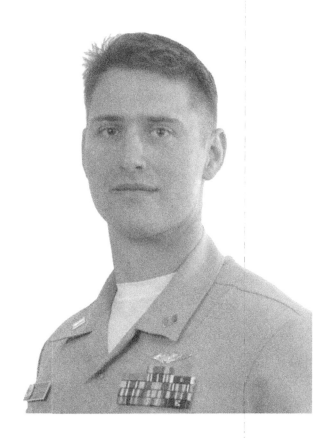

**KETTLEBELL EXERCISES BUILD WILL AND DISCIPLINE!
TWO NECESSARY TRAITS FOR BUILDING MENTAL TOUGHNESS.**

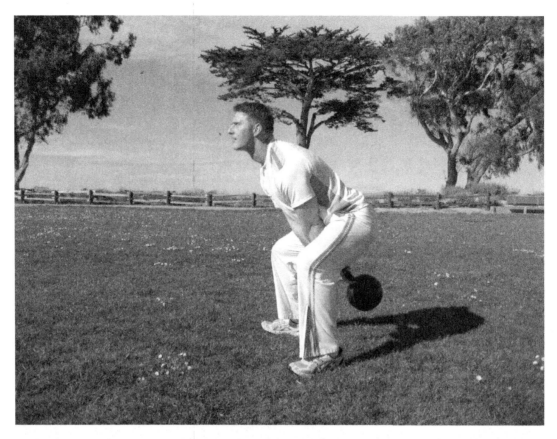

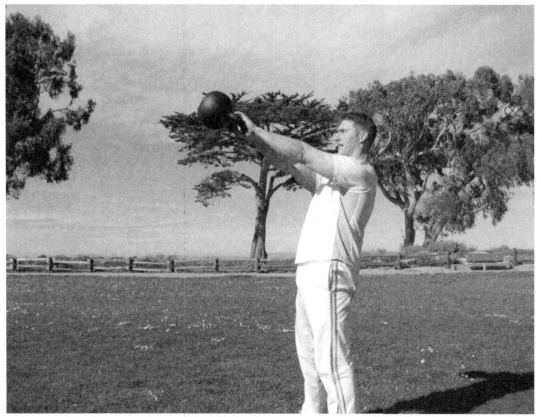

TWO HAND SWING

1. Place the kettlebell between your feet.

2. Sit back and without looking down let your hands slide down to grab the kettlebell.

3. Looking straight ahead and keeping your back flat raise the kettlebell off the ground.

4. Swing the kettlebell and exhale forcefully as you thrust your hips forward and squeeze your butt cheeks as if trying to pinch a penny with your glutes.

5. Power comes from the body, not the arms, the arms are hooks attached to the kettlebell.

6. Let the kettlebell swing down and inhale forcefully when the kettlebell passes your navel area.

7. Exhale forcefully and swing the kettlebell as described in step 4.

Note: 15 swings per 30 seconds is a good number to shoot for. When we are training for an event, me and my training partner count the number of swings and try to "beat" each other or set the bar at a higher standard, which usually means 18-20 swings per 30 seconds. Those three to five extra swings may not seem like much when you read them on paper, but you have to hump to get them in!

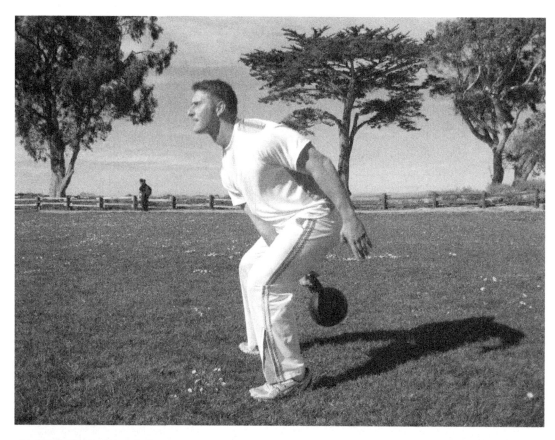

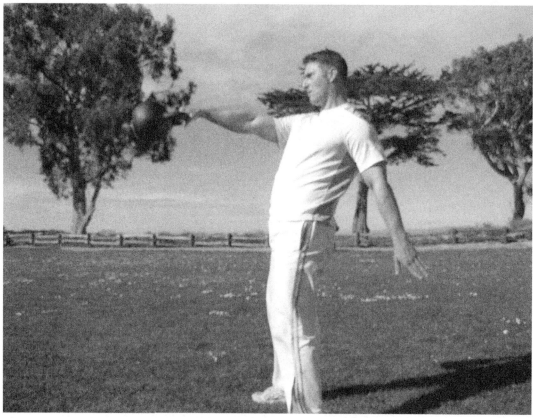

ONE HAND SWING

1. Place the kettlebell between your feet.

2. Sit back and without looking down let your hand slide down to grab the kettlebell.

3. Looking straight ahead and keeping your back flat raise the kettlebell off the ground.

4. Swing the kettlebell and exhale forcefully as you thrust your hips forward and squeeze your butt cheeks as if trying to pinch a penny with your glutes.

5. Power comes from the body, not the arms, the arms are hooks attached to the kettlebell.

6. Let the kettlebell swing down and inhale forcefully when the kettlebell passes your navel area.

7. Exhale forcefully and swing the kettlebell as described in step 4.

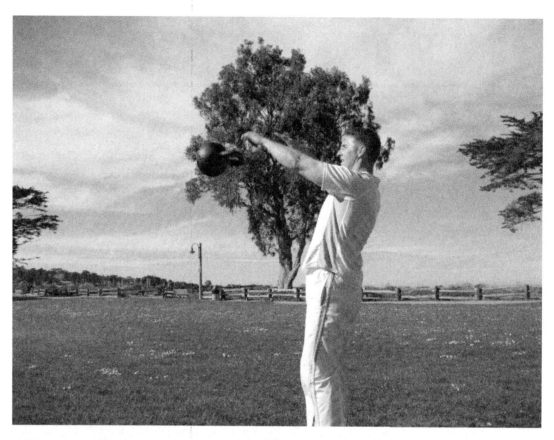

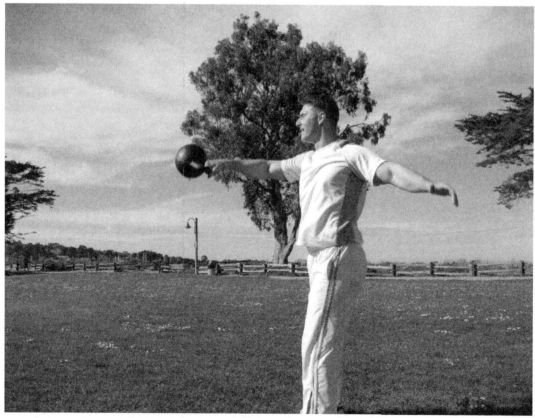

ALTERNATING ONE HAND SWING

1. Place the kettlebell between your feet.

2. Sit back and without looking down let your hand slide down to grab the kettlebell.

3. Looking straight ahead and keeping your back flat raise the kettlebell off the ground.

4. Swing the kettlebell and exhale forcefully as you thrust your hips forward and squeeze your butt cheeks as if trying to pinch a penny with your glutes. Really explode your hips forward.

5. Power comes from the body, not the arms, the arms are hooks attached to the kettlebell. Project your hip power into the kettlebell so that it will hang in midair in what is called "the float", the point where the upward swing is about to become downward.

6. Switch hands in "the float" of the swing.

7. Let the kettlebell swing down and inhale forcefully when the kettlebell passes your navel area.

8. Exhale forcefully and swing the kettlebell as described in step 4.

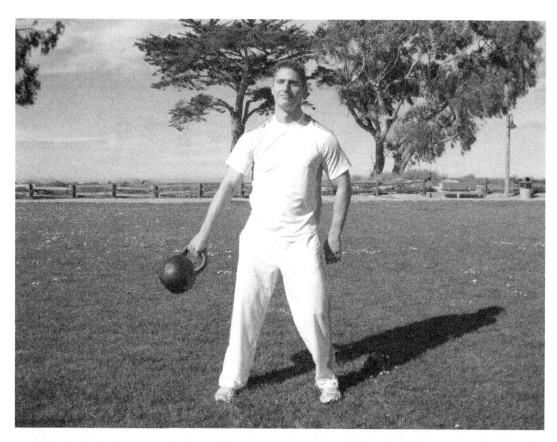

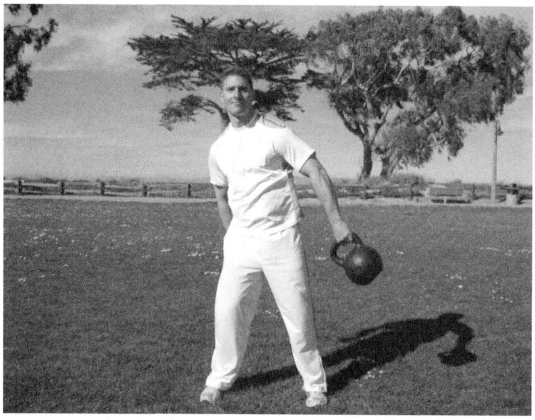

ROUND THE BODY
PASS

1.   Stand shoulder width apart.

2.   Swing the kettlebell in a circular fashion and pass from one hand to the other.

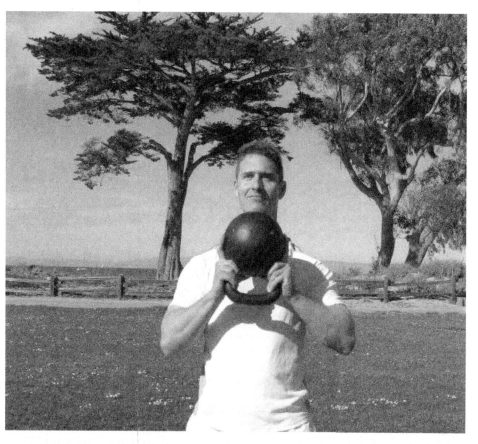

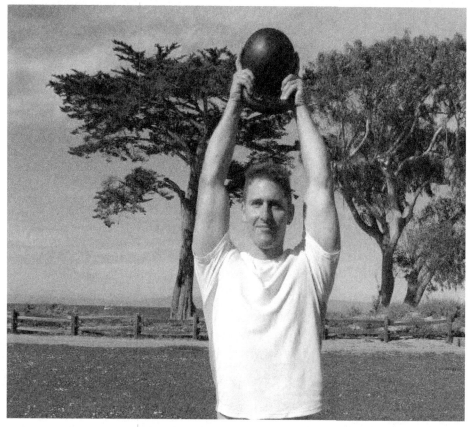

PRESS

1. Stand shoulder width apart with kettlebell between your feet.

2. Grab the kettlebell by the horns and press overhead.

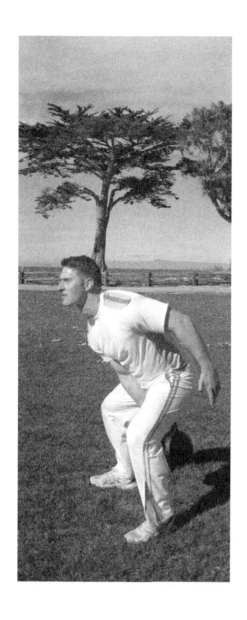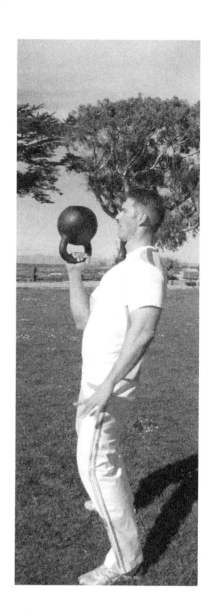

BOTTOMS UP

CLEAN

1. Stand with feet shoulder width apart with the kettlebell in between your feet.

2. Swing the kettlebell upward with the bottom facing up.

3. Hold the kettlebell in the bottoms up position at the top of the movement, squeeze hard, keep your elbow tight to your body, and squeeze the forearm of the free arm simultaneously.

4. Let the kettlebell swing back down and repeat.

5. The trick is to find the balance point. You can do it.

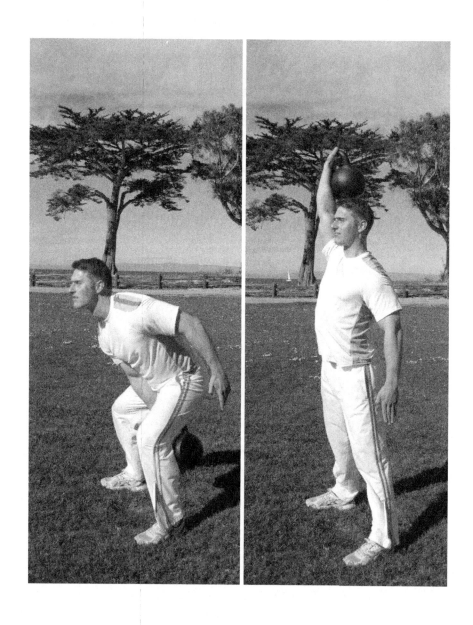

SNATCH

1. Stand with feet shoulder width apart and the kettlebell between your legs.

2. Sit back as you inhale while looking forward.

3. Forcefully exhale as you thrust your hips forward and squeeze your buttcheecks.

4. There are two ways to get to the top of the movement. The hardstyle approach is to punch up through the kettlebell as it reaches shoulder. This places the kettlebell on your forearm. The other approach is to open your hand and swing the kettlebell around it as you are coming to the top of the movement. This will place the kettlebell on your forearm. Refer to the DVD to SEE both of these techniques in action. Try both variations and see which one you prefer. Hold for one second once you get here with your arm locked.

5. There are two ways you can come down from the top movement. One is to simply swing it down. The other is to drop it to shoulder level, pause and then swing down from this halfway point. Try both variations and see which one you prefer. Refer to the DVD to SEE both of these in action.

Note: with the snatch aim for 10-12 repetitions for every 30 seconds.

"HOW YOUR DREAMS COME TRUE ISN'T AS IMPORTANT AS THE STRENGTH WITH WHICH YOU GRIP THEM."

-PETER RAGNAR

WEEK 1

This is your introduction to Extreme Military Fitness and is meant to allow you the opportunity to learn the exercises without taxing the body too much. Focus on good form over reps as you are battling against time, not a set number of repetitions. Go slow on the squat and drive your butt back to begin the movement. The knees should not be over the toes for this particular squat.

With the slo-mo squat aim for 3 complete repetitions in one minute. Here, less is more. With the slo-mo pushup take your time to learn proper form. This means that the elbows face towards your legs throughout all the movement. Avoid flaring your elbows to the side, since all this does is put undue stress on the chest and shoulder joint by forcing you to contract from a stretched position.

The Rope Crunch will hit your upper abs and the Bent Leg Jacknife will hit your lower abs. The key to doing the easy burpee and a lot of this program is the BREATHING. Let me repeat that the key to doing the burpee and a lot of this program is the BREATHING. Match the breathing pattern and work on good form rather than speed on this first week.

This week will also have you learning how to use the kettlebell. Recommended weights are 24lb for women and 35lb for men. The swing is the foundation exercise for the majority of the kettlebell exercises. I will let you know right now that you probably won't get the bottoms up clean the first workout. Treat it as skill practice until you get it. The way to do kettlebell circuits is six exercises for 30 seconds each. This makes a three minute round. You only have to do three rounds this first week. Enjoy it while it lasts.

WORKOUT 1

Slo-Mo Squats
Do 3 Sets of 1 Minute
Rest 1 Minute Between Sets

Slo-Mo Pushups
Do 3 Sets of 1 Minute
Rest 1 Minute Between Sets

Rope Crunch
Do 3 Sets of 1 Minute
Rest 1 Minute Between Sets

Easy Burpee
Do 3 Sets of 1 Minute
Rest 1 Minute Between Sets

WORKOUT 2

**Perform each exercise for 30 seconds in consecutive fashion until circuit is complete.
Take 1 minute rest in between circuits.**

Circuit 1
Two Hand Swing
Round the Body Pass
One Hand Swing
Round the Body Pass
One Hand Swing
Press

Circuit 2
Alternating One Arm Swing
Round the Body Pass
Bottoms Up Clean
Round the Body Pass
Bottoms Up Clean
Press

Circuit 3
Two Hand Swing
Round the Body
One Hand Swing
Round the Body
One Hand Swing
Press

WORKOUT 3

Slo-Mo Squats
Do 3 Sets of 1 Minute
Rest 1 Minute Between Sets

Slo-Mo Pushups
Do 3 Sets of 1 Minute
Rest 1 Minute Between Sets

Bent Leg Jacknife
Do 3 Sets of 1 Minute
Rest 1 Minute Between Sets

Easy Burpee
Do 3 Sets of 1 Minute
Rest 1 Minute Between Sets

WORKOUT 4

**Perform each exercise for 30 seconds in consecutive fashion until circuit is complete.
Take 1 minute rest in between circuits.**

Circuit 1
Two Hand Swing
Round the Body Pass
One Hand Swing
Round the Body Pass
One Hand Swing
Press

Circuit 2
Alternating One Arm Swing
Round the Body Pass
Bottoms Up Clean
Round the Body Pass
Bottoms Up Clean
Press

Circuit 3
Two Hand Swing
Round the Body
One Hand Swing
Round the Body
One Hand Swing
Press

"LIVE YOUR LIFE AS IF ALL YOUR DREAMS HAVE COME TRUE AND CHALLENGE REALITY TO CATCH UP."

-PETER THOMPSON

WEEK 2

This week your squats go up to two minutes, but other than that you keep on working on the foundation you were building the first week. By the end of this week you should be able to do the easy burpee fairly well.

The kettlebell circuits build on the foundation of week one and by the end of this week you should be able to do the bottoms up clean.

WORKOUT 5

Slo-Mo Squats
Do 3 Sets of 2 Minutes
Rest 1 Minute Between Sets

Slo-Mo Pushups
Do 3 Sets of 1 Minute
Rest 1 Minute Between Sets

Rope Crunch
Do 3 Sets of 1 Minute
Rest 1 Minute Between Sets

Easy Burpee
Do 3 Sets of 1 Minute
Rest 1 Minute Between Sets

WORKOUT 6

**Perform each exercise for 30 seconds in consecutive fashion until circuit is complete.
Take 1 minute rest in between circuits.**

Circuit 1
Two Hand Swing
Round the Body Pass
One Hand Swing
Round the Body Pass
One Hand Swing
Press

Circuit 2
Alternating One Arm Swing
Round the Body Pass
Bottoms Up Clean
Round the Body Pass
Bottoms Up Clean
Press

Circuit 3
Two Hand Swing
Round the Body
One Hand Swing
Round the Body
One Hand Swing
Press

WORKOUT 7

Slo-Mo Squats
Do 3 Sets of 2 Minutes
Rest 1 Minute Between Sets

Slo-Mo Pushups
Do 3 Sets of 1 Minute
Rest 1 Minute Between Sets

Bent Leg Jacknife
Do 3 Sets of 1 Minute
Rest 1 Minute Between Sets

Easy Burpee
Do 3 Sets of 1 Minute
Rest 1 Minute Between Sets

WORKOUT 8

**Perform each exercise for 30 seconds in consecutive fashion until circuit is complete.
Take 1 minute rest in between circuits.**

Circuit 1
Two Hand Swing
Round the Body Pass
One Hand Swing
Round the Body Pass
One Hand Swing
Press

Circuit 2
Alternating One Arm Swing
Round the Body Pass
Bottoms Up Clean
Round the Body Pass
Bottoms Up Clean
Press

Circuit 3
Two Hand Swing
Round the Body
One Hand Swing
Round the Body
One Hand Swing
Press

"THE REWARD FOR PRACTICE IS MORE PRACTICE."

-MATT FUREY

WEEK 3

OK, since you are starting to get conditioned you are going to do four sets of squats and four sets of pushups instead of the three you were doing in the last two weeks.

Now you are doing four kettlebell circuits and you are learning the snatch. Again, you have time to practice the snatch as the 30 seconds are not to get as many reps in as you can. Treat the time allotted as skill practice time until you get it right. Look at the instructions and pictures to get the motion. It is a fairly simple movement, yet it requires practice to get it down right. The snatch has been called the most powerful expression of the human body in kettlebell circles. Master this move and find out why. The snatch will become a staple of your kettlebell training in coming weeks, learn to love it.

WORKOUT 9

Slo-Mo Squats
Do 4 Sets of 2 Minutes
Rest 1 Minute Between Sets

Slo-Mo Pushups
Do 4 Sets of 1 Minute
Rest 1 Minute Between Sets

Rope Crunch
Do 3 Sets of 1 Minute
Rest 1 Minute Between Sets

Easy Burpee
Do 3 Sets of 1 Minute
Rest 1 Minute Between Sets

WORKOUT 10

**Perform each exercise for 30 seconds in consecutive fashion until circuit is complete.
Take 1 minute rest in between circuits.**

Circuit 1
Two Hand Swing
Round the Body Pass
One Hand Swing
Round the Body Pass
One Hand Swing
Press

Circuit 2
Alternating One Arm Swing
Round the Body Pass
Bottoms Up Clean
Round the Body Pass
Bottoms Up Clean
Press

Circuit 3
Snatch Right
Snatch Left
Round the Body Pass
Snatch Right
Snatch Left
Round the Body Pass

Circuit 4
Two Hand Swing
Round the Body
One Hand Swing
Round the Body
One Hand Swing
Press

WORKOUT 11

Slo-Mo Squats
Do 4 Sets of 2 Minutes
Rest 1 Minute Between Sets

Slo-Mo Pushups
Do 4 Sets of 1 Minute
Rest 1 Minute Between Sets

Bent Leg Jacknife
Do 3 Sets of 1 Minute
Rest 1 Minute Between Sets

Easy Burpee
Do 3 Sets of 1 Minute
Rest 1 Minute Between Sets

WORKOUT 12

**Perform each exercise for 30 seconds in consecutive fashion until circuit is complete.
Take 1 minute rest in between circuits.**

Circuit 1
Two Hand Swing
Round the Body Pass
One Hand Swing
Round the Body Pass
One Hand Swing
Press

Circuit 2
Alternating One Arm Swing
Round the Body Pass
Bottoms Up Clean
Round the Body Pass
Bottoms Up Clean
Press

Circuit 3
Snatch Right
Snatch Left
Round the Body Pass
Snatch Right
Snatch Left
Round the Body Pass

Circuit 4
Two Hand Swing
Round the Body
One Hand Swing
Round the Body
One Hand Swing
Press

"WE MUST REMEMBER THAT ONE MAN IS MUCH THE SAME AS ANOTHER, AND THAT HE IS BEST WHO IS TRAINED IN THE SEVEREST SCHOOL"

-THUCYDIDES

WEEK 4

Your bodyweight workouts remain the same so you can adapt to the increased workload.

Your kettlebell workouts for this week allow you to master the snatch and keep on building your endurance.

WORKOUT 13

Slo-Mo Squats
Do 4 Sets of 2 Minutes
Rest 1 Minute Between Sets

Slo-Mo Pushups
Do 4 Sets of 1 Minute
Rest 1 Minute Between Sets

Rope Crunch
Do 3 Sets of 1 Minute
Rest 1 Minute Between Sets

Easy Burpee
Do 3 Sets of 1 Minute
Rest 1 Minute Between Sets

WORKOUT 14

**Perform each exercise for 30 seconds in consecutive fashion until circuit is complete.
Take 1 minute rest in between circuits.**

Circuit 1
Two Hand Swing
Round the Body Pass
One Hand Swing
Round the Body Pass
One Hand Swing
Press

Circuit 2
Alternating One Arm Swing
Round the Body Pass
Bottoms Up Clean
Round the Body Pass
Bottoms Up Clean
Press

Circuit 3
Snatch Right
Snatch Left
Round the Body Pass
Snatch Right
Snatch Left
Round the Body Pass

Circuit 4
Two Hand Swing
Round the Body
One Hand Swing
Round the Body
One Hand Swing
Press

WORKOUT 15

Slo-Mo Squats
Do 4 Sets of 2 Minutes
Rest 1 Minute Between Sets

Slo-Mo Pushups
Do 4 Sets of 1 Minute
Rest 1 Minute Between Sets

Bent Leg Jacknife
Do 4 Sets of 1 Minute
Rest 1 Minute Between Sets

Easy Burpee
Do 4 Sets of 1 Minute
Rest 1 Minute Between Sets

WORKOUT 16

**Perform each exercise for 30 seconds in consecutive fashion until circuit is complete.
Take 1 minute rest in between circuits.**

Circuit 1
Two Hand Swing
Round the Body Pass
One Hand Swing
Round the Body Pass
One Hand Swing
Press

Circuit 2
Alternating One Arm Swing
Round the Body Pass
Bottoms Up Clean
Round the Body Pass
Bottoms Up Clean
Press

Circuit 3
Snatch Right
Snatch Left
Round the Body Pass
Snatch Right
Snatch Left
Round the Body Pass

Circuit 4
Two Hand Swing
Round the Body
One Hand Swing
Round the Body
One Hand Swing
Press

"IF THIS STRUGGLE IS ORDAINED OF US, WHY NOT ENTER IT WITH KINGLY COURAGE, WITH DAUNTLESS DELIGHT?"

-RAGNAR REDBEARD

WEEK 5

Welcome to month two of training! Now we step it up a notch and go into full squats and pushups. Strive to do as many as you can in good form. Instead of rope crunches and bent leg jackknife now you will do the more challenging needle lift and bicycle crunch for abs. You move away from the easy burpee and now call the burpee with pushup your regular staple for bodyweight workouts

This week also has you stepping it up a notch with the kettlebells as you will complete five circuits and two of those circuits will be "snatch-centric", meaning that you will focus on the snatch.

WORKOUT 17

Squats
Do 3 Sets of 2 Minutes
Rest 1 Minute Between Sets

Pushups
Do 3 Sets of 1 Minute
Rest 1 Minute Between Sets

Needle Lift
Do 3 Sets of 1 Minute
Rest 1 Minute Between Sets

Burpee with Pushup
Do 3 Sets of 1 Minute
Rest 1 Minute Between Sets

WORKOUT 18

**Perform each exercise for 30 seconds in consecutive fashion until circuit is complete.
Take 1 minute rest in between circuits.**

Circuit 1
Two Hand Swing
Round the Body Pass
One Hand Swing
Round the Body Pass
One Hand Swing
Press

Circuit 2
Alternating One Arm Swing
Round the Body Pass
Bottoms Up Clean
Round the Body Pass
Bottoms Up Clean
Press

Circuit 3
Snatch Right
Snatch Left
Round the Body Pass
Snatch Right
Snatch Left
Round the Body Pass

Circuit 4
Snatch Right
Alternating One Arm Swing
Round the Body Pass
Snatch Left
Alternating One Arm Swing
Round the Body Pass

Circuit 5
Two Hand Swing
Round the Body
One Hand Swing
Round the Body
One Hand Swing
Press

WORKOUT 19

Squats
Do 3 Sets of 2 Minutes
Rest 1 Minute Between Sets

Pushups
Do 3 Sets of 1 Minute
Rest 1 Minute Between Sets

Bicycle Situp
Do 3 Sets of 1 Minute
Rest 1 Minute Between Sets

Burpee with Pushup
Do 3 Sets of 1 Minute
Rest 1 Minute Between Sets

WORKOUT 20

**Perform each exercise for 30 seconds in consecutive fashion until circuit is complete.
Take 1 minute rest in between circuits.**

Circuit 1
Two Hand Swing
Round the Body Pass
One Hand Swing
Round the Body Pass
One Hand Swing
Press

Circuit 2
Alternating One Arm Swing
Round the Body Pass
Bottoms Up Clean
Round the Body Pass
Bottoms Up Clean
Press

Circuit 3
Snatch Right
Snatch Left
Round the Body Pass
Snatch Right
Snatch Left
Round the Body Pass

Circuit 4
Snatch Right
Alternating One Arm Swing
Round the Body Pass
Snatch Left
Alternating One Arm Swing
Round the Body Pass

Circuit 5
Two Hand Swing
Round the Body
One Hand Swing
Round the Body
One Hand Swing
Press

"HOW DO YOU BECOME ENTHUSIASTIC? ONLY DO THINGS THAT EXCITE YOU, ACTIONS THAT YOU ARE ENTHUSIASTIC ABOUT DOING, TASKS THAT AREN'T WORK BUT SIMPLY AN EXTENSION OF A LIFELONG PLAY TIME."

-PETER THOMPSON

WEEK 6

Here you ingrain into your body and nervous systems the new skills and level of conditioning you started working on in week 5 by practice, practice, practice.

WORKOUT 21

Squats
Do 3 Sets of 2 Minutes
Rest 1 Minute Between Sets

Pushups
Do 3 Sets of 1 Minute
Rest 1 Minute Between Sets

Needle Lift
Do 3 Sets of 1 Minute
Rest 1 Minute Between Sets

Burpee with Pushup
Do 3 Sets of 1 Minute
Rest 1 Minute Between Sets

WORKOUT 22

Perform each exercise for 30 seconds in consecutive fashion until circuit is complete.
Take 1 minute rest in between circuits.

Circuit 1
Two Hand Swing
Round the Body Pass
One Hand Swing
Round the Body Pass
One Hand Swing
Press

Circuit 2
Alternating One Arm Swing
Round the Body Pass
Bottoms Up Clean
Round the Body Pass
Bottoms Up Clean
Press

Circuit 3
Snatch Right
Snatch Left
Round the Body Pass
Snatch Right
Snatch Left
Round the Body Pass

Circuit 4
Snatch Right
Alternating One Arm Swing
Round the Body Pass
Snatch Left
Alternating One Arm Swing
Round the Body Pass

Circuit 5
Two Hand Swing
Round the Body
One Hand Swing
Round the Body
One Hand Swing
Press

WORKOUT 23

Squats
Do 3 Sets of 2 Minutes
Rest 1 Minute Between Sets

Pushups
Do 3 Sets of 1 Minute
Rest 1 Minute Between Sets

Bicycle Situp
Do 3 Sets of 1 Minute
Rest 1 Minute Between Sets

Burpee with Pushup
Do 3 Sets of 1 Minute
Rest 1 Minute Between Sets

WORKOUT 24

**Perform each exercise for 30 seconds in consecutive fashion until circuit is complete.
Take 1 minute rest in between circuits.**

Circuit 1
Two Hand Swing
Round the Body Pass
One Hand Swing
Round the Body Pass
One Hand Swing
Press

Circuit 2
Alternating One Arm Swing
Round the Body Pass
Bottoms Up Clean
Round the Body Pass
Bottoms Up Clean
Press

Circuit 3
Snatch Right
Snatch Left
Round the Body Pass
Snatch Right
Snatch Left
Round the Body Pass

Circuit 4
Snatch Right
Alternating One Arm Swing
Round the Body Pass
Snatch Left
Alternating One Arm Swing
Round the Body Pass

Circuit 5
Two Hand Swing
Round the Body
One Hand Swing
Round the Body
One Hand Swing
Press

"IF YOU ARE GOING TO TAKE VIENNA, TAKE VIENNA!"

- NAPOLEON

WEEK 7

That's right, we up the intensity again by adding one set to the squats and pushups for four sets total. The rest remains the same.

WORKOUT 25

Squats
Do 4 Sets of 2 Minutes
Rest 1 Minute Between Sets

Pushups
Do 4 Sets of 1 Minute
Rest 1 Minute Between Sets

Needle Lift
Do 3 Sets of 1 Minute
Rest 1 Minute Between Sets

Burpee with Pushup
Do 3 Sets of 1 Minute
Rest 1 Minute Between Sets

WORKOUT 26

**Perform each exercise for 30 seconds in consecutive fashion until circuit is complete.
Take 1 minute rest in between circuits.**

Circuit 1
Two Hand Swing
Round the Body Pass
One Hand Swing
Round the Body Pass
One Hand Swing
Press

Circuit 2
Alternating One Arm Swing
Round the Body Pass
Bottoms Up Clean
Round the Body Pass
Bottoms Up Clean
Press

Circuit 3
Snatch Right
Snatch Left
Round the Body Pass
Snatch Right
Snatch Left
Round the Body Pass

Circuit 4
Snatch Right
Alternating One Arm Swing
Round the Body Pass
Snatch Left
Alternating One Arm Swing
Round the Body Pass

Circuit 5
Two Hand Swing
Round the Body
One Hand Swing
Round the Body
One Hand Swing
Press

WORKOUT 27

Squats
Do 4 Sets of 2 Minutes
Rest 1 Minute Between Sets

Pushups
Do 4 Sets of 1 Minute
Rest 1 Minute Between Sets

Bicycle Situp
Do 3 Sets of 1 Minute
Rest 1 Minute Between Sets

Burpee with Pushup
Do 3 Sets of 1 Minute
Rest 1 Minute Between Sets

WORKOUT 28

**Perform each exercise for 30 seconds in consecutive fashion until circuit is complete.
Take 1 minute rest in between circuits.**

Circuit 1
Two Hand Swing
Round the Body Pass
One Hand Swing
Round the Body Pass
One Hand Swing
Press

Circuit 2
Alternating One Arm Swing
Round the Body Pass
Bottoms Up Clean
Round the Body Pass
Bottoms Up Clean
Press

Circuit 3
Snatch Right
Snatch Left
Round the Body Pass
Snatch Right
Snatch Left
Round the Body Pass

Circuit 4
Snatch Right
Alternating One Arm Swing
Round the Body Pass
Snatch Left
Alternating One Arm Swing
Round the Body Pass

Circuit 5
Two Hand Swing
Round the Body
One Hand Swing
Round the Body
One Hand Swing
Press

"THUS PROPERLY UNDERSTOOD, DARWINISM IS NOT A VERY COMFORTING DOCTRINE FOR FAT MEN."

- RAGNAR REDBEARD

WEEK 8

Whoa! What's happening here? Back to slow-mo squats and pushups and only three sets of each? Only four kettlebell circuits?

Here you are given a slight breather to recharge and attack the last month with intensity. By the end of this week you should feel hungry for more and recuperate physically and mentally for the last and final push.

WORKOUT 29

Slo-Mo Squats
Do 3 Sets of 1 Minutes
Rest 1 Minute Between Sets

Slo-Mo Pushups
Do 3 Sets of 1 Minute
Rest 1 Minute Between Sets

Needle Lift
Do 3 Sets of 1 Minute
Rest 1 Minute Between Sets

Burpee with Pushup
Do 3 Sets of 1 Minute
Rest 1 Minute Between Sets

WORKOUT 30

**Perform each exercise for 30 seconds in consecutive fashion until circuit is complete.
Take 1 minute rest in between circuits.**

Circuit 1
Two Hand Swing
Round the Body Pass
One Hand Swing
Round the Body Pass
One Hand Swing
Press

Circuit 2
Alternating One Arm Swing
Round the Body Pass
Bottoms Up Clean
Round the Body Pass
Bottoms Up Clean
Press

Circuit 3
Snatch Right
Snatch Left
Round the Body Pass
Snatch Right
Snatch Left
Round the Body Pass

Circuit 4
Two Hand Swing
Round the Body
One Hand Swing
Round the Body
One Hand Swing
Press

WORKOUT 31

Slo-Mo Squats
Do 3 Sets of 1 Minutes
Rest 1 Minute Between Sets

Slo-Mo Pushups
Do 3 Sets of 1 Minute
Rest 1 Minute Between Sets

Rope Crunch
Do 3 Sets of 1 Minute
Rest 1 Minute Between Sets

Burpee with Pushup
Do 3 Sets of 1 Minute
Rest 1 Minute Between Sets

WORKOUT 32

**Perform each exercise for 30 seconds in consecutive fashion until circuit is complete.
Take 1 minute rest in between circuits.**

Circuit 1
Two Hand Swing
Round the Body Pass
One Hand Swing
Round the Body Pass
One Hand Swing
Press

Circuit 2
Snatch Right
Snatch Left
Round the Body Pass
Snatch Right
Snatch Left
Round the Body Pass

Circuit 3
Two Hand Swing
Round the Body
One Hand Swing
Round the Body
One Hand Swing
Press

"WHAT ONE GREAT THING WOULD YOU DARE
TO DREAM IF YOU KNEW YOU COULD NOT
FAIL?"

-BRIAN TRACY

WEEK 9

After the dip in intensity last week you should be craving to hit it hard this week. Say no more, your wish has been granted! Now we will attack ABC squats and pushups. If you have ever lifted weights and heard of 21's, where you do 7 reps to from top of the movement to the middle, then 7 reps from the bottom of the movement to the middle and then finish with 7 full reps, then you know what is in store for you. You will do a similar arrangement for your squats and pushups. Yes, you WILL feel the burn! Love it! Now you are doing a burpee with jump to develop more conditioning and explosive power in your legs. Again the key lies in the BREATHING.

You must approach the kettlebell circuit with the attitude of "it was for THIS that I was training for" as you will do five circuits and three of them will be "snatch-centric".

WORKOUT 33

ABC Squats
Do 3 Sets of 2 Minutes
Rest 1 Minute Between Sets

ABC Pushups
Do 3 Sets of 1 Minute
Rest 1 Minute Between Sets

Bicycle Situp
Do 3 Sets of 1 Minute
Rest 1 Minute Between Sets

Burpee with Jump
Do 3 Sets of 1 Minute
Rest 1 Minute Between Sets

WORKOUT 34

Perform each exercise for 30 seconds in consecutive fashion until circuit is complete.
Take 1 minute rest in between circuits.

Circuit 1
Two Hand Swing
Round the Body Pass
One Hand Swing
Round the Body Pass
One Hand Swing
Press

Circuit 2
Alternating One Arm Swing
Round the Body Pass
Bottoms Up Clean
Round the Body Pass
Bottoms Up Clean
Press

Circuit 3
Snatch Right
Snatch Left
Round the Body Pass
Snatch Right
Snatch Left
Round the Body Pass

Circuit 4
Snatch Right
Alternating One Arm Swing
Round the Body Pass
Snatch Left
Alternating One Arm Swing
Round the Body Pass

Circuit 5
Snatch Right
Two Hand Swing
Round the Body Pass
Snatch Left
Two Hand Swing
Round the Body Pass

WORKOUT 35

ABC Squats
Do 3 Sets of 2 Minutes
Rest 1 Minute Between Sets

ABC Pushups
Do 3 Sets of 1 Minute
Rest 1 Minute Between Sets

Needle Lift
Do 3 Sets of 1 Minute
Rest 1 Minute Between Sets

Burpee with Jump
Do 3 Sets of 1 Minute
Rest 1 Minute Between Sets

WORKOUT 36

**Perform each exercise for 30 seconds in consecutive fashion until circuit is complete.
Take 1 minute rest in between circuits.**

Circuit 1
Two Hand Swing
Round the Body Pass
One Hand Swing
Round the Body Pass
One Hand Swing
Press

Circuit 2
Alternating One Arm Swing
Round the Body Pass
Bottoms Up Clean
Round the Body Pass
Bottoms Up Clean
Press

Circuit 3
Snatch Right
Snatch Left
Round the Body Pass
Snatch Right
Snatch Left
Round the Body Pass

Circuit 4
Snatch Right
Alternating One Arm Swing
Round the Body Pass
Snatch Left
Alternating One Arm Swing
Round the Body Pass

Circuit 5
Snatch Right
Two Hand Swing
Round the Body Pass
Snatch Left
Two Hand Swing
Round the Body Pass

"DISAPPOINTMENTS SEEM TO OCCUR MORE OFTEN WHEN WE EXPECT MORE FROM OTHERS THAN WE DO OF OURSELVES."

- PETER RAGNAR

WEEK 10

Here you work on refining your technique with the ABC squats, the burpees, the snatches, and the new level of conditioning that is being demanded from your body. Remember to focus on form and that the key lies in the BREATHING.

WORKOUT 37

ABC Squats
Do 3 Sets of 2 Minutes
Rest 1 Minute Between Sets

ABC Pushups
Do 3 Sets of 1 Minute
Rest 1 Minute Between Sets

Bicycle Situp
Do 3 Sets of 1 Minute
Rest 1 Minute Between Sets

Burpee with Jump
Do 3 Sets of 1 Minute
Rest 1 Minute Between Sets

WORKOUT 38

Perform each exercise for 30 seconds in consecutive fashion until circuit is complete. Take 1 minute rest in between circuits.

Circuit 1
Two Hand Swing
Round the Body Pass
One Hand Swing
Round the Body Pass
One Hand Swing
Press

Circuit 2
Alternating One Arm Swing
Round the Body Pass
Bottoms Up Clean
Round the Body Pass
Bottoms Up Clean
Press

Circuit 3
Snatch Right
Snatch Left
Round the Body Pass
Snatch Right
Snatch Left
Round the Body Pass

Circuit 4
Snatch Right
Alternating One Arm Swing
Round the Body Pass
Snatch Left
Alternating One Arm Swing
Round the Body Pass

Circuit 5
Snatch Right
Two Hand Swing
Round the Body Pass
Snatch Left
Two Hand Swing
Round the Body Pass

WORKOUT 39

ABC Squats
Do 3 Sets of 2 Minutes
Rest 1 Minute Between Sets

ABC Pushups
Do 3 Sets of 1 Minute
Rest 1 Minute Between Sets

Needle Lift
Do 3 Sets of 1 Minute
Rest 1 Minute Between Sets

Burpee with Jump
Do 3 Sets of 1 Minute
Rest 1 Minute Between Sets

WORKOUT 40

**Perform each exercise for 30 seconds in consecutive fashion until circuit is complete.
Take 1 minute rest in between circuits.**

Circuit 1
Two Hand Swing
Round the Body Pass
One Hand Swing
Round the Body Pass
One Hand Swing
Press

Circuit 2
Alternating One Arm Swing
Round the Body Pass
Bottoms Up Clean
Round the Body Pass
Bottoms Up Clean
Press

Circuit 3
Snatch Right
Snatch Left
Round the Body Pass
Snatch Right
Snatch Left
Round the Body Pass

Circuit 4
Snatch Right
Alternating One Arm Swing
Round the Body Pass
Snatch Left
Alternating One Arm Swing
Round the Body Pass

Circuit 5
Snatch Right
Two Hand Swing
Round the Body Pass
Snatch Left
Two Hand Swing
Round the Body Pass

"Fortes Fortuna Juvat!"
(Fortune Favors the Brave)

- Latin Proverb

WEEK 11

This week you stay the course and work on mastering the exercises and conditioning requirements that you started on this third month of your training.

WORKOUT 41

ABC Squats
Do 3 Sets of 2 Minutes
Rest 1 Minute Between Sets

Clockwork Pushups
Do 3 Sets of 1 Minute
Rest 1 Minute Between Sets

Bicycle Situp
Do 3 Sets of 1 Minute
Rest 1 Minute Between Sets

Burpee with Jump
Do 3 Sets of 1 Minute
Rest 1 Minute Between Sets

WORKOUT 42

Perform each exercise for 30 seconds in consecutive fashion until circuit is complete.
Take 1 minute rest in between circuits.

Circuit 1
Two Hand Swing
Round the Body Pass
One Hand Swing
Round the Body Pass
One Hand Swing
Press

Circuit 2
Alternating One Arm Swing
Round the Body Pass
Bottoms Up Clean
Round the Body Pass
Bottoms Up Clean
Press

Circuit 3
Snatch Right
Snatch Left
Round the Body Pass
Snatch Right
Snatch Left
Round the Body Pass

Circuit 4
Snatch Right
Alternating One Arm Swing
Round the Body Pass
Snatch Left
Alternating One Arm Swing
Round the Body Pass

Circuit 5
Snatch Right
Two Hand Swing
Round the Body Pass
Snatch Left
Two Hand Swing
Round the Body Pass

WORKOUT 43

ABC Squats
Do 3 Sets of 2 Minutes
Rest 1 Minute Between Sets

Clockwork Pushups
Do 3 Sets of 1 Minute
Rest 1 Minute Between Sets

Needle Lift
Do 3 Sets of 1 Minute
Rest 1 Minute Between Sets

Burpee with Jump
Do 3 Sets of 1 Minute
Rest 1 Minute Between Sets

WORKOUT 44

Perform each exercise for 30 seconds in consecutive fashion until circuit is complete.
Take 1 minute rest in between circuits.

Circuit 1
Two Hand Swing
Round the Body Pass
One Hand Swing
Round the Body Pass
One Hand Swing
Press

Circuit 2
Alternating One Arm Swing
Round the Body Pass
Bottoms Up Clean
Round the Body Pass
Bottoms Up Clean
Press

Circuit 3
Snatch Right
Snatch Left
Round the Body Pass
Snatch Right
Snatch Left
Round the Body Pass

Circuit 4
Snatch Right
Alternating One Arm Swing
Round the Body Pass
Snatch Left
Alternating One Arm Swing
Round the Body Pass

Circuit 5
Snatch Right
Two Hand Swing
Round the Body Pass
Snatch Left
Two Hand Swing
Round the Body Pass

"REFUSE TO MAKE EXCUSES OR BLAME ANYONE FOR ANYTHING."

-BRIAN TRACY

WEEK 12

This is it! The home stretch. To build more explosiveness we are going to do jump squats during this week. At this stage you should have mastered all the exercises and should aim for 100% intensity during the time allotted. One minute may not seem like much, but it IS when you are giving it your all. Remember, you are going to get out of this as much as you put in, so don't hold back or pace yourself. Find out what you can do and honor that United States Marine Corps credo "Pain is weakness leaving the body."

You can do it!

WORKOUT 45

Jump Squats
Do 3 Sets of 1 Minutes
Rest 1 Minute Between Sets

ABC Pushups
Do 3 Sets of 1 Minute
Rest 1 Minute Between Sets

Rope Crunch
Do 3 Sets of 1 Minute
Rest 1 Minute Between Sets

Burpee with Jump
Do 3 Sets of 1 Minute
Rest 1 Minute Between Sets

WORKOUT 46

**Perform each exercise for 30 seconds in consecutive fashion until circuit is complete.
Take 1 minute rest in between circuits.**

Circuit 1
Two Hand Swing
Round the Body Pass
One Hand Swing
Round the Body Pass
One Hand Swing
Press

Circuit 2
Alternating One Arm Swing
Round the Body Pass
Bottoms Up Clean
Round the Body Pass
Bottoms Up Clean
Press

Circuit 3
Snatch Right
Snatch Left
Round the Body Pass
Snatch Right
Snatch Left
Round the Body Pass

Circuit 4
Snatch Right
Alternating One Arm Swing
Round the Body Pass
Snatch Left
Alternating One Arm Swing
Round the Body Pass

Circuit 5
Snatch Right
Two Hand Swing
Round the Body Pass
Snatch Left
Two Hand Swing
Round the Body Pass

WORKOUT 47

Jump Squats
Do 3 Sets of 1 Minute
Rest 1 Minute Between Sets

Clockwork Pushups
Do 3 Sets of 1 Minute
Rest 1 Minute Between Sets

Knee Tucks
Do 3 Sets of 1 Minute
Rest 1 Minute Between Sets

Burpee with Jump
Do 3 Sets of 1 Minute
Rest 1 Minute Between Sets

WORKOUT 48

Perform each exercise for 30 seconds in consecutive fashion until circuit is complete.
Take 1 minute rest in between circuits.

Circuit 1
Two Hand Swing
Round the Body Pass
One Hand Swing
Round the Body Pass
One Hand Swing
Press

Circuit 2
Alternating One Arm Swing
Round the Body Pass
Bottoms Up Clean
Round the Body Pass
Bottoms Up Clean
Press

Circuit 3
Snatch Right
Snatch Left
Round the Body Pass
Snatch Right
Snatch Left
Round the Body Pass

Circuit 4
Snatch Right
Alternating One Arm Swing
Round the Body Pass
Snatch Left
Alternating One Arm Swing
Round the Body Pass

Circuit 5
Snatch Right
Two Hand Swing
Round the Body Pass
Snatch Left
Two Hand Swing
Round the Body Pass

A NOTE ON NUTRITION

While a complete nutritional regimen for 12 weeks is beyond the scope of this program, I am going to share with you one of my secret weapons regarding nutrition. It is my morning super foods shake.

The following is my super food shake:

1-2 fruits (bananas, strawberries, etc) – healthy carbohydrates and live enzymes
Distilled water – best medium for the super shake
1 packet Emergen-C – anti-oxidant
1-2 tablespoon flaxseeds – anti-estrogen
1 tablespoon maca – promotes testosterone in men and progesterone in women
2 tablespoons lecithin granules – supports brain function
1 teaspoon creatine (pure creatine only) – supports muscle activity
1 tablespoon bee pollen granules (raw and local is best) – chock full of nutrition
1 tablespoon raw local unheated honey – great against allergies and highly nutritious
¼ teaspoon raw Ginseng powder – qi tonic and adaptogen
20-30 grams protein powder or 3-4 raw eggs, (raw fertile eggs preferred)

Put it all in a blender and enjoy! You may want to start out with a teaspoon instead of a tablespoon for the above foods until you get used to them.

Chase it with one tablespoon of Omega-3 Fish Oils to further nourish the brain.

If you start drinking this super shake in the morning you will probably notice that you are not hungry until noon. This is because your body is being fed at a cellular level.

I used to eat cereal with rice milk and noticed that I was hungry one hour and a half after eating and would frequently eat some fruit or have a tuna fish sandwich.

With the shakes I just drank water until it was time to eat my lunch. I made the shake for my wife and she reported the same thing.

Try it faithfully for one month and let me know what you think! If you are like me then you can never go back and breakfast HAS to be a super shake.

Noted health pioneer Bernard Jensen considered adding four alfalfa tablets to every meal "almost a panacea". I don't know about you, but for about $14 for 1,000 tablets its worth a try. Let me know if it works for you, at least it will keep you regular.

Which brings us to our next subject…

A NOTE ON TRAINING YOUR WILL

If you want to become stronger physically and mentally to overcome any challenge in life, whether it be gutting out that last fifth kettlebell circuit or enduring whatever life throws at you, then you need mental toughness.

You need to train your mind and will to obey you and not succumb to weakness, desire or laziness.

One great way to do that is to go on a modified fast once a week, or once a month if that suits you better in the beginning, and eat nothing but water and three super shakes for that day.

Fasting trains your mind and willpower to do something slightly uncomfortable. If you have never done this I guarantee you that at the end of the day your thoughts will be very different than your regular thoughts. You will probably find yourself looking at books in your library you hadn't considered, getting new insights derived from deep thought and building confidence in yourself and your ability to honor your commitments.

Using the super shakes guarantees that you will get all the nutrition your body needs to be properly nourished, and gives the digestive system a day of rest.

The real stoics do water fasting, and while I believe that to be a worthwhile practice at the right time, it is not the most ideal during periods of heavy training. Another approach is juice fasting, which I have also done, but is not the most ideal when engaged in this type of training.

Give it an honest try for some or all of the 12 weeks and let me know how the process goes for you as well as the person you feel yourself becoming.

Now you have all the tools to become the man or woman you have always wanted to be.

When do you think is the best time to start this program and forge the new you?

F.A.Q.

Can I wear gloves for the kettlebell workouts?

In some circles they say that no self-respecting kettlebell lifter would wear gloves. I personally don't wear gloves and I am proud of the calluses I have earned. With that said if you feel gloves are preferable over calluses I have no objection and you have my blessing. Swing and snatch to your heart's content with gloved hands! I would remove all rings from your hands before using a kettlebell though.

What is the checklist method that you refer to?

If you look at the instructions for each exercise you will notice that they are in numbered fashion. The easiest way is to convert the instructions into a single word or command and then just run the exercise "by the numbers" or what we call the checklist method. For example you might reduce the snatch to "Swing, Punch, Lock, Drop." Same can be applied to the burpee, the Easy Burpee can be "Squat, Kick, Tuck, Stand" or any other word choice that reminds you to do ALL the steps in the movement. The greatest mistake people make is "cutting corners" when they are learning a new movement. It goes something like this "Oh I know he said something about punching it thru for a snatch but I am just going to try and swing it all the way up." Make a checklist of ALL the steps and do ALL the steps. This is the checklist method.

What do we do for warmup?

Nothing really, these routines make the first set the warmup set, after which you start upping the intensity. Since these are all functional exercises they warmup the body as you go. What this really means is to concentrate on FORM over speed during the first set, not only to warmup, but to set the correct mental groove of how the exercise is to be performed during that workout. Once you have laid the correct performance tracks in your mind for the first set, then see what you can do by aiming for higher number of reps in the next sets.

I am having problems with the burpee, what do I do?

Treat the exercise as learning a SKILL and forget about the number of reps, focus exclusively on FORM even if you only get 5 repetition for the time allotted. The way to do this is to follow the checklist method and GO AT YOUR OWN PACE. When practicing burpees just make sure to hit all the steps: "Squat, Kick, Tuck, Stand" and make sure to incorporate PROPER BREATHING into it as well. Yes, if you have not worked out in a while it can be challenging, but you can master it, even if you are 50, and you do not need to go at my pace from the DVD to get the benefit from this exercise.

How do you work out with your training partner?

While you can do everything here solo it works best when you have a training partner. The way I like to do it is to have my training partner task me with the the exercises in the circuit every 30 seconds via verbal commands. What you want to do is free your mind and put all your focus on the exercise. If you are completely open and receptive to your partner's commands then you just PERFORM. Trust me, I can do the circuits with a lot more intensity when I just LISTEN to a command and EXECUTE than when I am looking at a piece of paper and a timekeeping device to see what exercise comes next. Plus let's not forget the good old factor of competition. You can start counting the number of repetitions you and your partner do per time period and try to beat each other or set a standard that you will not deviate from. When you know you are being held accountable you will perform that much better.

Your burpee method slows me down, I can do them faster, but can't because you want me to do all these steps and breathe a certain way.

OK, while this is not a question it is a common complaint from the guys with a higher level of conditioning. Here is the "trick" to it. While EVERYONE needs to learn how to do it right at first marking all the steps and matching each step with either an inhale or an exhale, at the advanced levels you do multiple moves per inhale or exhale. For example when I do jump burpees here is MY breathing pattern. 1. INHALE – Squat, 2. EXHALE – Kick legs out, push down to ground, push back up to plank position, 3 – INHALE – Tuck legs in ready to spring up, 4 EXHALE – Spring up as high as I can. Again the key is learning to meter your breath, have a clean and crisp matching of breath to movements and learning to RELAX.

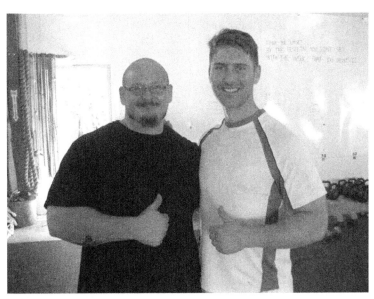

I want to thank Bud Jeffries for believing in me and my course.
May it help you achieve awesome levels of fitness!

Printed in Great Britain
by Amazon

29146767R00079